Vegan Soup: Delicious Vegan Soup Recipes for Better Health and Easy Weight Loss

by **Alissa Noel Grey**
Text copyright(c)2014 Alissa Noel Grey

CW01497330

Table Of Contents

Heartwarming Vegan Soups for all Seasons and Tastes

Soups are fast, light and warming, they are also nourishing, healing and soothing when prepared in the right way. Homemade vegan soups make a great meal, either as a as a healthy lunch, weeknight dinner or even for the festive season get-togethers.

In my family we simply love soup and I prepare one every day. We even sometimes have soup for breakfast because soup only needs reheating and it is easily digestible yet nourishing. Prepared at home from your own vegetables and legumes, vegan soups are incredibly filling and will not make you hungry a few hours later either.

The vegan soups I am offering you in my new cookbook have been handed down from generation to generation over the years and I have personally tasted them all. They have been slightly adapted to suit our and our kids' tastes and they are always absolutely delicious, healthy and budget friendly.

Creamy Broccoli and Potato Soup

Serves: 4-5

Prep time: 30 min

Ingredients:

3 cups broccoli, cut into florets and chopped

2 potatoes, peeled and chopped

1 large onion, chopped

3 garlic cloves, minced

1 cup raw cashews

1 cup vegetable broth

4 cups water

3 tbsp extra virgin olive oil

1/2 tsp ground nutmeg

Directions:

Soak cashews in a bowl covered with water for at least 4 hours. Drain water and blend cashews with 1 cup of vegetable broth until smooth. Set aside.

Gently heat olive oil in a large saucepan over medium-high heat. Cook onion and garlic and for 3-4 minutes until tender. Add in broccoli, potato, nutmeg and water.

Cover and bring to the boil, then reduce heat and simmer for 20 minutes, stirring from time to time. Remove from heat and stir in cashew mixture.

Blend until smooth, return to pan and cook until heated through.

Creamy Brussels Sprout Soup

Serves: 4-5

Prep time: 30 min

Ingredients:

1 lb frozen Brussels sprouts, thawed

2 potatoes, peeled and chopped

1 large onion, chopped

3 garlic cloves, minced

1 cup raw cashews

4 cups vegetable broth

3 tbsp extra virgin olive oil

1/2 tsp curry powder

salt and black pepper, to taste

Directions:

Soak cashews in a bowl covered with water for at least 4 hours. Drain water and blend cashews with 1 cup of vegetable broth until smooth. Set aside.

Gently heat olive oil in a large saucepan over medium-high heat. Cook onion and garlic and for 3-4 minutes until tender. Add in Brussels sprouts, potato, curry and vegetable broth.

Cover and bring to a boil, then reduce heat and simmer for 20 minutes, stirring from time to time. Remove from heat and stir in cashew mixture.

Blend until smooth, return to pan and cook until heated through.

Creamy Potato Soup

Serves: 4-5

Prep time: 35 min

Ingredients:

6 medium potatoes, cut into small cubes

1 leek, white part only, chopped

1 carrot, chopped

1 zucchini, peeled and chopped

1 celery stalk, chopped

3 cups water

1 cup coconut milk

3 tbsp extra virgin olive oil

salt and black pepper, to taste

Directions:

Gently heat olive oil in a deep saucepan and sauté the onion for 2-3 minutes. Add in potatoes, carrot, zucchini and celery and cook for 2-3 minutes, stirring.

Add in water and salt and bring to a boil, then lower heat and simmer until the vegetables are tender.

Blend until smooth, add coconut milk, blend some more and serve.

Leek, Brown Rice and Potato Soup

Serves: 4-5

Prep time: 35 min

Ingredients:

3 potatoes, peeled and diced

2 leeks, finely chopped

1/4 cup brown rice

5 cups water

3 tbsp extra virgin olive oil

lemon juice, to taste

Directions:

Heat olive oil in a deep soup pot and sauté leeks for 3-4 minutes. Add in potatoes and cook for a minute more. Stir in water, bring to a boil, and the brown rice.

Reduce heat and simmer for 30 minutes. Add lemon juice, to taste, and serve.

Turnip and Potato Soup

Serves 4-5

Prep time: 30 min

Ingredients:

1 onion, chopped

2 garlic cloves, minced

2 cups, diced potatoes

2 cups diced turnip

1 cup chopped kale

3 cups vegetable broth

1 cup coconut milk

3 tbsp extra virgin olive oil

1/2 tsp dried thyme

salt, to taste

black pepper, to taste

Directions:

Gently heat olive oil in a large saucepan over medium-high heat. Cook onion and garlic for 3-4 minutes until tender.

Add turnips, potatoes and the broth. Season with salt and black pepper to taste. Sprinkle with thyme and bring to a boil. Cover and simmer for 20 minutes or until the potato and turnip are tender.

Stir in the kale and the coconut milk and allow to simmer together another 2-3 minutes.

Italian Cabbage Soup

Serves: 4-5

Prep time: 45 min

Ingredients:

1 onion, chopped

1/2 head cabbage, shredded

1 carrot, chopped

1 potato, peeled and diced

1 celery stalk, sliced

1 can (15 oz) diced tomatoes, undrained

3 cups vegetable broth

1 tsp Italian seasoning

3 tbsp extra virgin olive oil

salt and pepper, to taste

Directions:

Heat the oil over medium heat and gently sauté the onion until translucent. Add in cabbage, carrot, potato, celery, tomatoes and seasoning and stir to combine.

Add in the broth, bring the soup to a boil, reduce heat, and simmer for 30-35 minutes. Season with salt and black pepper to taste.

Mediterranean Chickpea Soup

Serves 4-5

Ingredients:

1 can (15 oz) chickpeas, drained

1 small onion, chopped

2 garlic cloves, minced

1 can (15 oz) tomatoes, diced

2 cups water

2 cups coconut milk

3 tbsp extra virgin olive oil

2 bay leaves

1/2 tsp dried oregano

Directions:

Heat olive oil in a deep soup pot and sauté onion and garlic for 1-2 minutes. Add in water, chickpeas, tomatoes, bay leaves, and oregano.

Bring the soup to a boil then reduce heat and simmer for 20 minutes. Add in coconut milk and cook for 1-2 minutes more. Set aside to cool, discard the bay leaves and blend until smooth.

Carrot, Sweet Potato and Chickpea Soup

Serves: 5-6

Prep time: 25 min

Ingredients:

3 large carrots, chopped

1/2 onion, chopped

1 can (15 oz) chickpeas, undrained

2 sweet potatoes, peeled and diced

4 cups vegetable broth

2 tbsp extra virgin olive oil

1 tsp cumin

1 tsp ginger

Directions:

Heat olive oil in a large saucepan over medium heat. Add onion and carrots and sauté until tender. Add in broth, chickpeas, sweet potato and seasonings.

Bring to a boil then reduce heat and simmer, covered, for 30 minutes. Blend soup until smooth, add coconut milk and cook for 2-3 minutes until heated through.

Sweet Potato and Coconut Soup

Serves: 4-5

Prep time: 25 min

Ingredients:

1 small onion, chopped

2 lb sweet potatoes, peeled and diced

4 cups vegetable broth

1 can coconut milk

2 tbsp extra virgin olive oil

1 tsp nutmeg

Directions:

Heat olive oil in a large saucepan over medium heat. Add onion and sauté until tender. Add in broth, sweet potato and nutmeg.

Bring to a boil then reduce heat and simmer, covered, for 30 minutes. Blend soup until smooth and cook for 2-3 minutes until heated through.

Creamy Tomato and Roasted Pepper Soup

Serves: 4-5

Prep time: 35 min

Ingredients:

1 (12-ounce) jar roasted red peppers, drained and chopped

1 large onion, chopped

2 garlic cloves, minced

4 medium tomatoes, chopped

4 cups vegetable broth

3 tbsp extra virgin olive oil

2 bay leaves

Directions:

Heat olive oil in a large saucepan over medium-high heat and sauté onion for 3-4 minutes, stirring. Add in garlic and sauté until just fragrant. Stir in the red peppers, bay leaves and tomatoes and simmer for 10 minutes.

Add broth, season with salt and pepper and bring to the boil. Reduce heat and simmer for 20 minutes. Set aside to cool slightly, remove the bay leaves and blend, in batches, until smooth.

Fresh Asparagus Soup

Serves: 4-5

Prep time: 35 min

Ingredients:

2 lb fresh asparagus, cut into ½-inch pieces.

1 large onion, chopped

2 garlic cloves, minced

½ cup raw cashews, soaked in warm water for 1 hour

3 cups vegetable broth

3 tbsp extra virgin olive oil

lemon juice, to taste

Directions:

Heat olive oil in a large saucepan over medium-high heat and sauté onion for 3-4 minutes, stirring. Add in garlic and sauté until just fragrant. Stir in asparagus and simmer for 5 minutes.

Add broth, season with salt and pepper and bring to the boil. Reduce heat and simmer for 20 minutes. Set aside to cool slightly, add cashews, and blend, in batches, until smooth. Season with lemon juice and serve.

Creamy Red Lentil Soup

Serves: 4-5

Prep time: 35 min

Ingredients:

1 cup red lentils

1/2 small onion, chopped

2 garlic cloves, chopped

1/2 red pepper, chopped

3 cups vegetable broth

1 cup coconut milk

3 tbsp extra virgin olive oil

1 tbsp paprika

1/2 tsp ginger

1 tsp cumin

salt and black pepper, to taste

Directions:

Gently heat olive oil in a large saucepan. Add onion, garlic, red pepper, paprika, ginger and cumin and sauté, stirring, until just fragrant. Add in red lentils and vegetable broth.

Bring to a boil, cover, and simmer for 15 minutes. Add in coconut milk and simmer for 5 more minutes. Remove from heat, season with salt and black pepper, and blend until smooth. Serve hot.

Lentil, Barley and Kale Soup

Serves: 4-5

Prep time: 35 min

Ingredients:

2 medium leeks, chopped

3 garlic cloves, chopped

2 bay leaves

1 can tomatoes (15 oz), diced and undrained

1/2 cup red lentils

1/2 cup barley

1 bunch kale (10 oz), stemmed and coarsely chopped

4 cups water

3 tbsp extra virgin olive oil

1 tsp paprika

½ tsp cumin

Directions:

Heat oil in a large saucepan over medium-high heat. Sauté leeks and garlic until just fragrant. Add cumin and paprika, tomatoes, lentils, barley, and water. Season with salt and pepper.

Cover and bring to the boil then reduce heat and simmer for 40 minutes or until barley is tender. Add in kale, stir it in, and let it simmer for five minutes more.

Mediterranean Lentil and Chickpea Soup

Serves: 4-5

Prep time: 20 min

Ingredients:

1 cup red lentils

2 carrots, chopped

1 onion, chopped

1 garlic clove, chopped

1 small red pepper, chopped

1 can tomatoes, chopped

½ can chickpeas, drained

½ can white beans, drained

1 celery stalk, chopped

6 cups water

1 tbsp paprika

1 tsp ginger, grated

1 tsp cumin

3 tbsp extra virgin olive oil

Directions:

Heat olive oil in a deep soup pot and gently sauté onions, garlic, red pepper and ginger.

Add in water, lentils, chickpeas, white beans, tomatoes, carrots, celery, and cumin.

Bring to a boil then lower heat and simmer for 20 minutes, or until the lentils are tender.

Purée half the soup in a food processor. Return the puréed soup to the pot, stir and serve.

Moroccan Carrot and Chickpea Soup

Serves: 4-5

Prep time: 20 min

Ingredients:

4 carrots, chopped

1 onion, chopped

1 garlic clove, minced

1 can chickpeas, undrained

4 cups vegetable broth

3-4 tbsp extra virgin olive oil

1 tsp paprika

1 tsp grated ginger

salt and black pepper, to taste

Directions:

Heat olive oil in a deep soup pot over medium-high heat. Gently sauté onion, garlic and carrots for 3-4 minutes, stirring. Add in paprika, ginger, broth and chickpeas.

Bring to the boil then reduce heat and simmer, covered, for 10 minutes. Blend soup until smooth and return to pan. Cook over medium-high heat until heated through. Season with salt and pepper to taste and serve.

Celery and Carrot Soup

Serves: 4-5

Prep time: 20 min

Ingredients:

2 celery stalks, chopped

1 large apple, chopped

1/2 onion, chopped

2 carrots, chopped

1 garlic clove, minced

4 cups vegetable broth

3-4 tbsp extra virgin olive oil

1 tsp paprika

1 tsp grated ginger

salt and black pepper, to taste

Directions:

Heat olive oil in a deep soup pot over medium-high heat. Gently sauté onion, garlic and carrots for 3-4 minutes, stirring. Add in paprika, ginger, celery, apple and broth.

Bring to the boil then reduce heat and simmer, covered, for 10 minutes. Blend soup until smooth and return to pan. Cook over medium-high heat until heated through.

Season with salt and pepper to taste and serve.

Pea, Dill and Rice Soup

Serves: 4

Prep time: 10 min

Ingredients:

1 (16 oz) bag frozen green peas

1 onion, chopped

3-4 garlic cloves, chopped

1/3 cup rice

3 tbsp fresh dill, chopped

3 tbsp extra virgin olive oil

fresh dill, finely chopped, to serve

salt and pepper, to taste

Directions:

Heat oil in a large saucepan over medium-high heat and sauté onion and garlic for 3-4 minutes.

Add in peas and vegetable broth and bring to the boil. Stir in rice, cover, reduce heat, and simmer for 15 minutes. Add dill, season with salt and pepper and serve sprinkled with fresh dill.

Minted Nettle & Pea Soup

Serves: 4

Prep time: 10 min

Ingredients:

1 onion, chopped

3-4 garlic cloves, chopped

4 cups vegetable broth

2 tbsp dried mint leaves

1 16 oz bag frozen green peas

about 20 nettle tops

3 tbsp extra virgin olive oil

fresh dill, finely chopped, to serve

Directions:

Heat oil in a large saucepan over medium-high heat and sauté onion and garlic for 3-4 minutes.

Add in dried mint, peas, washed nettles, and vegetable broth and bring to the boil. Cover, reduce heat, and simmer for 10 minutes.

Remove from heat and set aside to cool slightly, then blend in batches, until smooth. Return soup to saucepan over medium-low heat and cook until heated through. Season with salt and pepper. Serve sprinkled with fresh dill.

Bean and Pasta Soup

Serves: 4-5

Prep time: 10-15 min

Ingredients:

1 onion, chopped

2 large carrots, chopped

2 garlic cloves, minced

1 cup cooked orzo

1 15 oz can white beans, rinsed and drained

1 15 oz can tomatoes, diced and undrained

1 cup baby spinach leaves

3 cups water

1 tbsp paprika

1 tbsp dried mint

3 tbsp extra virgin olive oil

salt and black pepper, to taste

Directions:

Heat the olive oil over medium heat and gently sauté the onion, garlic and carrots. Add in tomatoes, water, salt and pepper, and bring to a boil.

Reduce heat and cook for 5-10 minutes, or until the carrots are tender. Stir in orzo, beans and spinach, and simmer until spinach is wilted.

Bean and Spinach Soup

Serves: 4-5

Prep time: 10-15 min

Ingredients:

1 onion, chopped

1 large carrot, chopped

2 garlic cloves, minced

1 15 oz can white beans, rinsed and drained

1 cup spinach leaves, trimmed and washed

3 cups vegetable broth

1 tbsp paprika

1 tbsp dried mint

3 tbsp extra virgin olive oil

salt and black pepper, to taste

Directions:

Heat the olive oil over medium heat and gently sauté the onion, garlic and carrot. Add in beans, broth, salt and pepper and bring to a boil.

Reduce heat and cook for 10 minutes, or until the carrots are tender. Stir in spinach, and simmer for about 5 minutes, until spinach is wilted.

Lima Bean Soup

Serves: 5-6

Prep time: 3-4 hrs for soaking, 120 min for cooking

Ingredients:

1 lb dry Lima beans

4-5 cups water

2 leeks, white part only, chopped

1 small onion, finely cut

1 celery stalk, chopped

3 carrots, chopped

5 cups vegetable broth

4 tbsp extra virgin olive oil

salt and black pepper, to taste

Directions:

Wash the Lima beans and soak them in water for a few hours. Discard the water, pour 3 cups of fresh water and cook the beans for an hour; discard this water too.

In a deep soup pot, heat olive oil and sauté the onion, leeks, celery and carrots until tender-crisp. Add 5 cups of vegetable broth and the Lima beans.

Stir, bring to the boil, lower heat and simmer for 1 hour. Season with salt and black pepper and purée half the soup in a food processor. Return the puréed soup to the pot, stir and serve.

Garden Vegetable Soup

Serves: 4-5

Prep time: 25 min

Ingredients:

2 leeks, white and pale green parts only, well rinsed and thinly sliced

1 large zucchini, peeled and diced

1 medium fennel bulb, trimmed, cored, and cut into large chunks

2 garlic cloves, chopped

3 cups vegetable broth

1 cup canned tomatoes, drained and chopped

1/2 cup vermicelli, broken into small pieces

3 tbsp extra virgin olive oil

black pepper, to taste

Directions:

Heat the olive oil in a large stockpot. Add the leeks and sauté over low heat for 5 minutes. Add in the zucchini, fennel and garlic and cook for about 5 minutes.

Stir in the vegetable broth and the tomatoes and bring to the boil. Reduce heat and simmer, uncovered, for 20 minutes, or until the vegetables are tender but still holding their shape. Stir in the vermicelli.

Simmer for a further 5 minutes and serve.

Spiced Beet and Carrot Soup

Serves: 4-5

Prep time: 25 min

Ingredients:

3 beets, washed and peeled

2 carrots, peeled and chopped

1 small onion, chopped

1 garlic clove, chopped

3 cups vegetable broth

1 cup water

2 tbsp extra virgin olive oil

1 tsp grated ginger

1 tsp grated orange peel

Directions:

Heat the olive oil in a large stockpot. Add the onion and sauté over low heat for 3-4 minutes or until translucent. Add the garlic, beets, carrots, ginger and lemon rind.

Stir in water and vegetable broth and bring to the boil. Reduce heat to medium and simmer, partially covered, for 30 minutes, or until beets are tender. Cool slightly and blend soup in batches until smooth. Season with salt and pepper and serve.

Simple White Bean Soup

Serves: 4-5

Prep time: 60 min

Ingredients:

1 cup white beans

1 carrot

1 onion, finely chopped

1 tomato, grated

1 red bell pepper, chopped

1 tbsp dried mint

1 tbsp paprika

2 tbsp extra virgin olive oil

salt, to taste

fresh parsley, chopped, to serve

Directions:

Soak the beans in cold water overnight. Rinse, drain and place in a deep soup pot. Cover the beans with cold water. Add in all remaining ingredients.

Bring to the boil and simmer until the beans are tender. Serve sprinkled with finely chopped parsley.

Garlicky Cauliflower Soup

Serves: 4-5

Prep time: 35 min

Ingredients:

1 medium head cauliflower, chopped

2 garlic cloves, minced

3 cups vegetable broth

1 cup coconut oil

3-4 tbsp extra virgin olive oil

salt, to taste

black pepper, to taste

Directions:

Heat the olive oil in a deep pot over medium heat and gently sauté the cauliflower for 4-5 minutes. Stir in the garlic and vegetable broth and bring to a boil.

Reduce heat, cover, and simmer for 30 minutes. Add in coconut milk and blend in a blender until smooth. Season with salt and pepper to taste and serve.

Creamy Pumpkin and Bell Pepper Soup

Serves: 4-5

Prep time: 35 min

Ingredients:

1/2 small onion, chopped

3 cups pumpkin cubes

2 red bell peppers, chopped

1 carrot, chopped

3 cups vegetable broth

3 tbsp extra virgin olive oil

1/2 tsp cumin

salt and black pepper, to taste

Directions:

Heat the olive oil in a deep soup pot and sauté the onion for 4-5 minutes. Add in the pumpkin, carrot and bell peppers and cook, stirring, for 5 minutes.

Stir in the broth and cumin and bring to the boil. Reduce heat to low, cover, and simmer, stirring occasionally, for 30 minutes, or until vegetables are soft.

Season with salt and pepper, blend in batches and reheat to serve.

Cream of Mushroom Soup

Serves: 4-5

Prep time: 35 min

Ingredients:

2 lbs mushrooms, peeled and chopped

1 large onion, chopped

2 garlic cloves, minced

3 cups vegetable broth

salt and pepper, to taste

3 tbsp extra virgin olive oil

Directions:

Sauté onions and garlic in a large soup pot until transparent. Add thyme and mushrooms.

Stir and cook for 10 minutes, then add the vegetable broth and simmer for another 10-20 minutes. Blend, season and serve.

Fast Mushroom and Kale Soup

Serves: 4-5

Prep time: 30 min

Ingredients:

1 onion, chopped

1 carrot, chopped

1 zucchini, peeled and diced

1 potato, peeled and diced

10 white mushrooms, chopped

1 bunch kale (10 oz), stemmed and coarsely chopped

3 cups vegetable broth

4 tbsp extra virgin olive oil

salt and black pepper. to taste

Directions:

Gently heat olive oil in a large soup pot. Add in onions, carrot and mushrooms and cook until vegetables are tender.

Stir in zucchini, kale and vegetable broth. Season to taste with salt and pepper and simmer for 20 minutes.

Spinach Soup

Serves: 4-5

Prep time: 35 min

Ingredients:

14 oz frozen spinach, slightly thawed

1 large onion, chopped

1 small carrot, chopped

1 small zucchini, peeled and chopped

3 cups hot water

4 tbsp extra virgin olive oil

1 tbsp paprika

salt and black pepper, to taste

Directions:

Heat oil in a deep cooking pot. Add in the onion and carrot and cook for 3-4 minutes, until tender. Add in paprika, spinach, zucchini and water and stir.

Season with salt and black pepper and bring to the boil. Reduce heat and simmer for around 30 minutes.

Homemade Lentil Soup

Serves: 4-5

Prep time: 35 min

Ingredients:

1 cup brown lentils

1 small onion, chopped

4 garlic cloves, minced

1 medium carrot, chopped

3 cups warm water

4 tbsp extra virgin olive oil

1 tbsp paprika

1 tbsp oregano

1/2 tsp salt

Directions:

Heat olive oil in a deep soup pot and cook the onions and carrots until tender. Add in paprika, garlic, lentils, oregano and water, stir, and bring to the boil.

Reduce heat and cook, covered, for 30 minutes. Add salt and simmer for 10 minutes more.

Italian-style Vegetable Minestrone

Serves: 4-5

Prep time: 25 min

Ingredients:

1/2 onion, chopped

2 garlic cloves, chopped

¼ cabbage, chopped

1 carrot, chopped

2 celery stalks, chopped

3 cups water

1 cup canned tomatoes, diced, undrained

1 1/2 cup green beans, trimmed and cut into 1/2-inch pieces

1/2 cup pasta, cooked

2-3 fresh basil leaves

2 tbsp extra virgin olive oil

black pepper and salt, to taste

Directions:

Heat the olive oil in a large pot over medium-high heat. Add the onion and cook until translucent, about 4 minutes. Add in the garlic, carrot and celery and cook for 5 minutes more.

Stir in the green beans, cabbage, tomatoes, basil, and water and bring to a boil. Reduce heat and simmer uncovered, for 15 minutes, or until vegetables are tender.

Stir in pasta, season with pepper and salt to taste and serve.

Lemon Artichoke Soup

Serves: 4-5

Prep time: 35 min

Ingredients:

3 cups artichoke hearts, chopped

1/2 onion, chopped

1 celery stalk, chopped

1 carrot, chopped

2 garlic cloves, minced

2 cups vegetable broth

2 tbsp olive oil

1 tsp salt

2 tbsp lemon juice

1 cup coconut milk

Directions:

Heat olive oil in a large pot and gently sauté the onion, celery, carrot, and garlic until the onion and garlic are translucent.

Stir in vegetable broth, artichokes and salt and bring to the boil. Reduce heat, add lemon juice and simmer for 15 minutes. Set aside to cool and blend until smooth. Stir in coconut milk and simmer for another 5 minutes.

Velvet Artichoke Hearts Soup

Serves: 4-5

Prep time: 35 min

Ingredients:

3 cups artichoke hearts, chopped

1/2 onion, chopped

2 celery stalk, chopped

1 small potato, peeled and chopped

2 garlic cloves, minced

2 cups vegetable broth

1 cup coconut milk

2 tbsp olive oil

1 tsp salt

black pepper, to serve

Directions:

Heat olive oil in a large pot and gently sauté the onion, celery and garlic until just fragrant. Stir in vegetable broth, coconut milk, artichokes and salt and bring to the boil.

Reduce heat and simmer for 15 minutes. Set aside to cool and blend until smooth. Serve sprinkled with black pepper.

Creamy Quinoa, Sweet Potato and Tomato Soup

Serves: 4

Prep time: 20 min

Ingredients:

½ cup quinoa

1 onion, chopped

1 large sweet potato, peeled and chopped

½ cup canned chickpeas, drained

1 cup baby spinach leaves

1 can tomatoes, drained and diced

3 cups vegetable broth

1 cup water

2 cloves garlic, chopped

1 tbsp grated fresh ginger

1 tsp cumin

1 tbsp paprika

2 tbsp extra virgin olive oil

Directions:

Wash quinoa very well, drain and set aside.

In a large soup pot, heat the olive oil over medium heat. Add the onions and garlic and sauté about 1-2 minutes, stirring. Add the sweet potato and sauté for another minute then add in the paprika, ginger and cumin.

Add water and broth, bring to a boil and stir in quinoa and tomatoes. Reduce heat to low, cover, and simmer about 15 minutes, or until the sweet potatoes are tender. Season with salt and black pepper to taste.

Blend the soup and return to the pot. Add the chickpeas and heat through, then add the spinach and cook until it wilts.

Leek and Quinoa Soup

Serves: 4-5

Prep time: 15 min

Ingredients:

½ cup quinoa

3 leeks, white part only, sliced

3 garlic cloves, chopped

1 potato, cut in small cubes

½ cup canned chickpeas, drained

4 cups vegetable broth

1 cup coconut milk

2 tbsp extra virgin olive oil

½ tsp ground coriander

1 tsp turmeric

salt and black pepper, to taste

Directions:

In a large soup pot, heat the olive oil over medium heat. Add the garlic and sauté for 1-2 minutes, stirring. Add the spices and stir.

Add the broth and bring to the boil then add in the quinoa, leeks, chickpeas and potato. Reduce heat and simmer, covered, for 15 minutes.

When the leeks are soft, add in a cup of coconut milk, stir, and simmer for 2 more minutes.

Red Lentil and Quinoa Soup

Serves: 4

Prep time: 20 min

Ingredients:

½ cup quinoa

1 cup red lentils

5 cups water

1 onion, chopped

2-3 garlic cloves, chopped

½ red bell pepper, finely cut

1 small tomato, chopped

3 tbsp extra virgin olive oil

1 tsp ginger

1 tsp cumin

1 tbsp paprika

salt and black pepper, to taste

Directions:

Wash and drain quinoa and red lentils and set aside.

In a large soup pot, heat the olive oil over medium heat. Add the onion, garlic and red pepper and sauté for 1-2 minutes, stirring. Add the paprika and spices and stir. Add in the red lentils and quinoa, stir and add the water.

Gently bring to the boil, then lower heat and simmer, covered for 15 minutes. Add the tomato and cook for five more minutes. Blend the soup and serve.

Spinach and Quinoa Soup

Serves: 4-5

Prep time: 20 min

Ingredients:

½ cup quinoa

1 onion, chopped

1 garlic clove, chopped

1 small zucchini, peeled and diced

1 tomato, diced

2 cups fresh spinach, cut

4 cups water

3 tbsp extra virgin olive oil

1 tbsp paprika

salt and pepper, to taste

Directions:

Heat olive oil in a deep soup pot over medium-high heat. Add onion and garlic and sauté for 1 minute, stirring constantly. Add in paprika and zucchini, stir, and cook for 2-3 minutes more.

Add 4 cups of water and bring to a boil then add in spinach and quinoa. Stir and reduce heat. Simmer for 15 minutes then set aside to cool.

Vegetable Quinoa Soup

Serves: 4-5

Prep time: 20 min

Ingredients:

½ cup quinoa

1 cup sliced leeks

1 garlic clove, chopped

½ carrot, diced

1 tomato, diced

1 small zucchini, diced

½ cup frozen green beans

4 cups water

1 tsp paprika

4 tbsp extra virgin olive oil

5-6 tbsp lemon juice, to serve

Directions:

Wash quinoa in a fine sieve under running water until the water runs clear. Set aside to drain.

Heat olive oil in a soup pot and gently sauté the leeks, garlic and carrot for 1 minute, stirring. Add paprika, zucchini, tomatoes, green beans and water.

Bring to a boil, add quinoa and lower heat to medium-low. Simmer for 15 minutes, or until the vegetables are tender. Serve with lemon juice.

Tomato and Quinoa Soup

Serves: 4-5

Prep time: 35 min

Ingredients:

4 cups chopped fresh tomatoes

1 onion, chopped

1/3 cup quinoa

2 cups water

1 garlic clove, minced

3 tbsp extra virgin olive oil

1 tbsp paprika

1 tsp salt

½ tsp black pepper

1 tbsp sugar

fresh parsley, chopped, to serve

Directions:

Heat olive oil in a large soup pot and sauté onions until translucent. Add in paprika, garlic and tomatoes and water and bring to the boil. Simmer for 10 minutes then blend the soup and return it to the pot.

Add the very well washed quinoa and a tablespoon of sugar and bring to the boil again. Simmer for 15 minutes stirring occasionally. Serve sprinkled with parsley.

Kale, Leek and Quinoa Soup

Serves: 4-5

Prep time: 35 min

Ingredients:

½ cup quinoa

2 leeks, white part only, chopped

1/2 onion, chopped

1 can tomatoes, diced and undrained

1 bunch kale (10 oz), stemmed and coarsely chopped

4 cups vegetable broth

3 tbsp extra virgin olive oil

salt and pepper, to taste

Directions:

Heat olive oil in a large pot over medium heat and gently sauté the onion for 3-4 minutes. Add in the leeks, season with salt and pepper and add the vegetable broth, tomatoes and quinoa.

Bring to a boil then reduce heat and simmer for 10 minutes. Stir in kale and cook for another 5 minutes.

FREE BONUS RECIPES: 20 Superfood Vegan Smoothies for Vibrant Health and Easy Weight Loss

Kale and Kiwi Smoothie

Serves: 2

Prep time: 2-3 min

Ingredients:

2-3 ice cubes

1 cup orange juice

1 small pear, peeled and chopped

2 kiwi, peeled and chopped

2-3 kale leaves

2-3 dates, pitted

Directions:

Combine all ingredients in a high speed blender and blend until smooth.

Delicious Broccoli Smoothie

Serves: 2

Prep time: 2-3 min

Ingredients:

2-3 frozen broccoli florets

1 cup coconut milk

1 banana, peeled and chopped

1 cup pineapple, cut

1 peach, chopped

1 tsp cinnamon

Directions:

Combine all ingredients in a high speed blender and blend until smooth.

Papaya Smoothie

Serves: 2

Prep time: 2-3 min

Ingredients:

2-3 frozen broccoli florets

1 cup orange juice

1 small ripe avocado, peeled, cored and diced

1 cup papaya

1 cup fresh strawberries

Directions:

Combine all ingredients in a high speed blender and blend until smooth.

Beet and Papaya Smoothie

Serves: 2

Prep time: 2-3 min

Ingredients:

3-4 ice cubes

1 cup orange juice

1 banana, peeled and chopped

1 cup papaya

1 small beet, peeled and cut

Directions:

Combine all ingredients in a high speed blender and blend until smooth.

Lean Green Smoothie

Serves: 2

Prep time: 2-3 min

Ingredients:

1 frozen banana, chopped

1 cup orange juice

2-3 kale leaves, stems removed

1 small cucumber, peeled and chopped

1/2 cup fresh parsley leaves

½ tsp grated ginger

Directions:

Combine all ingredients in a high speed blender and blend until smooth.

Easy Antioxidant Smoothie

Serves: 2

Prep time: 2-3 min

Ingredients:

2-3 frozen broccoli florets

1 cup orange juice

2 plums, cut

1 cup raspberries

1 tsp ginger powder

Directions:

Combine all ingredients in a high speed blender and blend until smooth.

Healthy Purple Smoothie

Serves: 2

Prep time: 2-3 min

Ingredients:

2-3 frozen broccoli florets

1 cup water

1/2 avocado, peeled and chopped

3 plums, chopped

1 cup blueberries

Directions:

Combine all ingredients in a high speed blender and blend until smooth.

Mom's Favorite Kale Smoothie

Serves: 2

Prep time: 2-3 min

Ingredients:

2-3 ice cubes

1½ cup orange juice

1 green small apple, cut

½ cucumber, chopped

2-3 leaves kale

½ cup raspberries

Directions:

Combine all ingredients in a high speed blender and blend until smooth.

Creamy Green Smoothie

Serves: 2

Prep time: 2-3 min

Ingredients:

1 frozen banana

1 cup coconut milk

1 small pear, chopped

1 cup baby spinach

1 cup grapes

1 tbsp coconut butter

1 tsp vanilla extract

Directions:

Combine all ingredients in a high speed blender and blend until smooth.

Strawberry and Arugula Smoothie

Serves: 2

Prep time: 2-3 min

Ingredients:

2 cups frozen strawberries

1 cup unsweetened almond milk

10-12 arugula leaves

1/2 tsp ground cinnamon

Directions:

Combine ice, almond milk, strawberries, arugula and cinnamon in a high speed blender. Blend until smooth and serve.

Emma's Amazing Smoothie

Serves: 2

Prep time: 2-3 min

Ingredients:

1 frozen banana, chopped

1 cup orange juice

1 large nectarine, sliced

1/2 zucchini, peeled and chopped

2-3 dates, pitted

Directions:

Combine all ingredients in a high speed blender and blend until smooth.

Good-To-Go Morning Smoothie

Serves: 2

Prep time: 2-3 min

Ingredients:

1 cup frozen strawberries

1 cup apple juice

1 banana, chopped

1 cup raw asparagus, chopped

1 tbsp ground flaxseed

Directions:

Combine all ingredients in a high speed blender and blend until smooth.

Endless Energy Smoothie

Serves: 2

Prep time: 2-3 min

Ingredients:

1 frozen banana, chopped

11/2 cup green tea

1 cup chopped pineapple

2 raw asparagus spears, chopped

1 lime, juiced

1 tbsp chia seeds

Directions:

Combine all ingredients in a high speed blender and blend until smooth.

High-fiber Fruit Smoothie

Serves: 2

Prep time: 2-3 min

Ingredients:

1 frozen banana, chopped

1 cup orange juice

2 cups chopped papaya

1 cup shredded cabbage

1 tbsp chia seeds

Directions:

Combine all ingredients in a high speed blender and blend until smooth.

Nutritious Green Smoothie

Serves: 2

Prep time: 2-3 min

Ingredients:

2-3 frozen broccoli florets

1 cup apple juice

1 large pear, chopped

1 kiwi, peeled and chopped

1 cup spinach leaves

1-2 dates, pitted

Directions:

Combine all ingredients in a high speed blender and blend until smooth.

Apricot, Strawberry and Banana Smoothie

Serves: 2

Prep time: 2-3 min

Ingredients:

1 frozen banana

11/2 cup almond milk

5 dried apricots

1 cup fresh strawberries

Directions:

Combine all ingredients in a high speed blender and blend until smooth.

Spinach and Green Apple Smoothie

Serves: 2

Prep time: 2-3 min

Ingredients:

3-4 ice cubes

1 cup unsweetened almond milk

1 banana, peeled and chopped

2 green apples, peeled and chopped

1 cup raw spinach leaves

3-4 dates, pitted

1 tsp grated ginger

Directions:

Combine all ingredients in a high speed blender and blend until smooth.

Superfood Blueberry Smoothie

Serves: 2

Prep time: 2-3 min

Ingredients:

2-3 cubes frozen spinach

1 cup green tea

1 banana

2 cups blueberries

1 tbsp ground flaxseed

Directions:

Combine all ingredients in a high speed blender and blend until smooth.

Zucchini and Blueberry Smoothie

Serves: 2

Prep time: 2-3 min

Ingredients:

1 cup frozen blueberries

1 cup unsweetened almond milk

1 banana

1 zucchini, peeled and chopped

Directions:

Combine all ingredients in a high speed blender and blend until smooth.

Tropical Spinach Smoothie

Serves: 2

Prep time: 2-3 min

Ingredients:

1/2 cup crushed ice or 3-4 ice cubes

1 cup coconut milk

1 mango, peeled and diced

1 cup fresh spinach leaves

4-5 dates, pitted

1/2 tsp vanilla extract

Directions:

Combine all ingredients in a high speed blender and blend until smooth.

About the Author

Alissa Noel Grey lives in a small French village in the foothills of a beautiful mountain range with her husband, three teenage kids, two free spirited dogs, and various other animals.

Alissa is incredibly lucky to be able to cook and eat natural foods, mostly grown nearby, something she's done since she was a teenager. She enjoys reading, hanging out with her family, going for long hikes, and growing organic vegetables and herbs.

25877230R00042

Printed in Great Britain
by Amazon